ATKINS DIET COOKBOOK

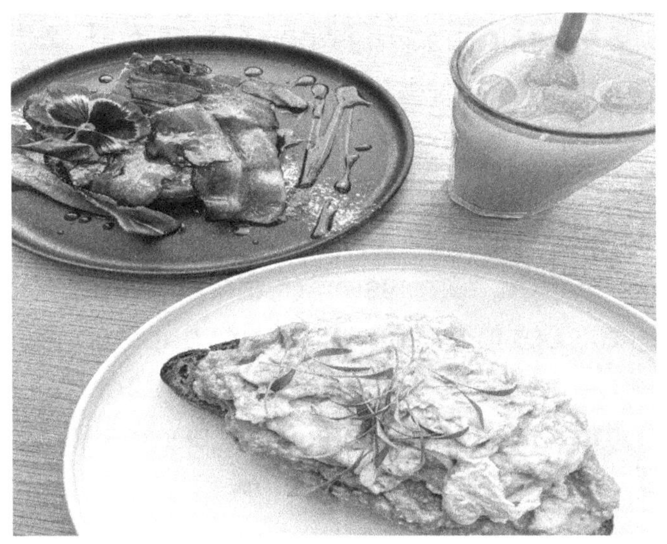

"Delicious Low-Carb Recipes for a Healthier You: A Comprehensive Guide to Mastering the Atkins Diet"

EMMA LYNCH

EMMA LYNCH
Copyright © 2023 by [Emma Lynch]

TABLE OF CONTENTS

INTRODUCTION

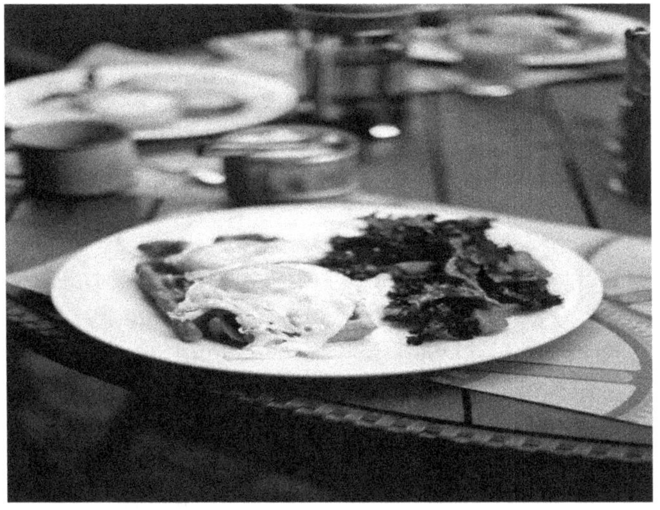

In the bustling rhythm of modern life, where time seems to slip away effortlessly, our relationship with food often becomes a balancing act between convenience and health. Imagine embarking on a journey where your meals not only energize you but also contribute to a profound transformation in your well-being. Allow me to share a brief story that could very well echo your own experiences.

Meet Sarah, a vibrant individual navigating the challenges of a busy lifestyle while harboring a desire for a healthier existence. Frustrated by fad diets that promised the moon but left her feeling unsatisfied and fatigued, Sarah discovered the Atkins Diet—a transformative approach that not only aligned with her nutritional goals but also embraced a realistic and sustainable perspective on eating.

This cookbook is an ode to Sarah's journey and to countless others who have embarked on a path of rejuvenation through the Atkins Diet. As we delve into the pages ahead, we'll explore a culinary adventure filled with delicious low-carb recipes designed to nourish the body, ignite taste buds, and foster a renewed sense of vitality.

So, join me as we embark on a flavorful expedition through the world of Atkins, where wholesome meals and mindful choices converge to create a lifestyle that transcends the limitations of traditional diets. Welcome to a culinary voyage that celebrates the joy of eating well and embraces the transformative power of the Atkins Diet.

BENEFITS OF FOLLOWING THE ATKINS DIET

The following are the benefits of following an Atkins diet:

1. **Weight Loss:**

- Atkins has been shown to be effective for weight loss, primarily due to the initial phase inducing ketosis, where the body burns stored fat for energy.

2. **Improved Blood Sugar Levels:**
   - The low-carb approach can help regulate blood sugar levels, making it beneficial for individuals with insulin resistance or type 2 diabetes.

3. **Increased Satiety:**
   - Consuming protein and healthy fats in the diet can lead to increased feelings of fullness and reduced hunger.

4. **Enhanced Energy Levels:**
   - Supporters of the Atkins Diet often report sustained energy levels throughout the day, avoiding the energy crashes associated with high-carb diets.

5. **Better Triglyceride and HDL Cholesterol Levels:**
   - Some studies suggest that the Atkins Diet may positively impact lipid profiles, improving triglyceride levels and increasing high-density lipoprotein (HDL) cholesterol.

6. **Reduced Inflammation:**
   - Lowering carbohydrate intake may contribute to a reduction in inflammatory markers, potentially benefiting individuals with inflammatory conditions.

7. **Improved Mental Clarity:**
   - Some individuals on the Atkins Diet report improved mental focus and clarity, possibly linked to stabilized blood sugar levels.

8. **Flexible and Sustainable:**
   - The phased approach allows for flexibility and personalization, making it easier for individuals to adopt the diet as a long-term lifestyle.

9. **Preservation of Lean Muscle Mass:**
   - Adequate protein intake in the diet helps preserve muscle mass during weight loss.

10. **Positive Effects on Metabolic Health:**
   - Some research suggests that low-carb diets, including Atkins, may have positive effects on various metabolic markers, such as insulin sensitivity.

It's important to note that individual responses to the Atkins Diet can vary, and consulting with a healthcare professional before making significant dietary changes is advisable. Additionally, long-term adherence to any diet should be approached with consideration for individual health needs and preferences.

CHAPTER ONE

GETTING STARTED

Getting started with the Atkins Diet involves several key steps:

1. **Educate Yourself:**
   - Understand the principles of the Atkins Diet, including the four phases and the emphasis on low-carb, high-fat, and adequate protein intake.

2. **Set Realistic Goals:**
   - Define your weight loss or health goals and establish a clear timeline. Keep in mind that the Atkins Diet is a gradual and phased approach.

3. **Clean Out Your Pantry:**
   - Remove high-carb and processed foods from your kitchen to create a supportive environment for your dietary changes.

4. **Plan Your Meals:**
   - Create a meal plan for the first week, focusing on low-carb, nutrient-dense foods. This helps you stay on track and avoid impulsive, high-carb choices.

5. **Stock Up on Essentials:**

- Ensure you have Atkins-friendly foods readily available, including lean proteins, healthy fats, low-carb vegetables, and suitable snacks.

6. **Hydration is Key:**
   - Drink plenty of water throughout the day to stay hydrated and help your body adapt to the dietary changes.

7. **Start with the Induction Phase:**
   - Begin with the Induction Phase, where carbohydrate intake is severely restricted to initiate ketosis. Follow the guidelines for allowable foods.

8. **Track Your Progress:**
   - Keep a food diary to monitor your daily intake and track your progress. This can help you identify patterns and make adjustments as needed.

9. **Incorporate Physical Activity:**
   - Include regular exercise in your everyday routine. It complements the Atkins Diet by supporting overall health and aiding in weight loss.

10. **Seek Support:**
    - Join online forums, find a buddy with similar goals, or involve family and friends for support. Having a community can be instrumental in staying motivated.

Remember, the Atkins Diet is a lifestyle change, and individual responses may vary. If you have existing health concerns, consult with a healthcare professional before making significant dietary changes.

UNDERSTANDING CARBOHYDRATES

Understanding carbohydrates is crucial for navigating the Atkins Diet effectively. Along with proteins and fats, carbohydrates are one of the three primary macronutrients. They are composed of sugar molecules and are classified into three types: sugars, starches, and fiber.

1. **Simple Carbohydrates (Sugars):**
   - Found in fruits, vegetables, and dairy products.
   - Also present in processed foods as added sugars (sucrose, glucose, fructose).

2. **Complex Carbohydrates (Starches):**
   - Rich in starchy vegetables, grains, and legumes.
   - Broken down into sugar during digestion.

3. **Dietary Fiber:**
   - present in whole grains, legumes, fruits, and vegetables.
   - Not fully digestible by the body, providing bulk to stool and promoting digestive health.

In the context of the Atkins Diet, understanding the concept of "net carbs" is essential. Net carbs are calculated by subtracting the dietary fiber content from the total carbohydrate content of a food item. The focus is on limiting net carbs to promote a state of ketosis, where the body burns fat for energy.

During the Atkins Diet phases:

- **Induction Phase:** Daily net carb intake is limited to 20-25 grams to initiate ketosis.

- **Balancing, Pre-Maintenance, and Maintenance Phases:** Carbohydrate intake is gradually increased while monitoring individual tolerance.

Foods allowed on the Atkins Diet typically include lean proteins, healthy fats, and low-carb vegetables. It's important to read food labels, choose whole, unprocessed foods, and be mindful of hidden sugars in various products.

Remember, individual responses to carbohydrates vary, and finding the right balance that works for your body is key. Consult with a healthcare professional or a registered dietitian for personalized advice, especially if you have underlying health conditions.

PHASES OF THE ATKINS DIET

The Atkins Diet is structured into four distinct phases, each serving a specific purpose in the overall approach to weight loss and lifestyle change:

1. **Induction Phase:**
   - **Objective:** Initiate ketosis for rapid fat burning and kickstart weight loss.
   - **Duration:** Typically 2 weeks but can be extended based on individual goals.
   - **Carbohydrate Intake:** Limited to 20-25 grams of net carbs per day, primarily from low-carb vegetables.
   - **Allowed Foods:** High-fat and moderate-protein foods, including meat, fish, eggs, butter, and oils.

2. **Balancing Phase:**
   - **Objective:** Gradually introduce more carbohydrates while continuing to lose weight.
   - **Duration:** Until you are within 10 pounds of your goal weight.
   - **Carbohydrate Intake:** Slowly increase net carbs, primarily from nuts, seeds, and low-carb vegetables.
   - **Allowed Foods:** Expands to include a wider variety of low-carb options, with continued emphasis on protein and healthy fats.

3. **Pre-Maintenance Phase:**

- **Objective:** Fine-tune carb intake to approach your goal weight.
  - **Duration:** When you are within 5-10 pounds of your goal weight.
  - **Carbohydrate Intake:** Gradually increase net carbs, incorporating more fruits, legumes, and whole grains.
  - **Allowed Foods:** Broadens to include a wider range of nutrient-dense carbohydrates while monitoring weight loss progress.

4. **Maintenance Phase:**
  - **Objective:** Sustain weight loss and a healthy lifestyle.
  - **Duration:** Ongoing.
  - **Carbohydrate Intake:** Establishes a personalized, sustainable level of net carbs that allows weight maintenance.
  - **Allowed Foods:** Adapts to individual tolerance, maintaining a balance between healthy carbs, proteins, and fats for a long-term approach.

It's essential to note that the transition between phases is gradual, allowing the body to adapt to changing carbohydrate levels. Individuals may progress through the phases at different rates based on their goals and responses to the diet. Always consult with a healthcare professional before starting any significant dietary changes.

SETTING PERSONAL GOALS

Setting personal goals is a crucial step in navigating the Atkins Diet. Here's a guide to help you establish meaningful and achievable objectives:

1. **Define Your Why:**
   - Clarify your motivation for following the Atkins Diet. Whether it's weight loss, improved health, increased energy, or other reasons, having a clear purpose enhances commitment.

2. **Be Specific:**
   - Clearly articulate your goals. Instead of a general aim like "lose weight," specify the amount of weight you want to lose and the timeframe in which you aim to achieve it.

3. **Consider Health Goals:**
   - Look beyond weight loss. Consider health-related goals such as improved blood sugar levels, increased energy, or better cholesterol profiles.

4. **Set Realistic Targets:**
   - Verify that you can complete your tasks within a suitable time frame. Unrealistic expectations can lead to frustration and discourage long-term commitment.

5. **Break Down Larger Goals:**

- If your ultimate goal is significant, break it into smaller, more manageable milestones. Honoring small victories along the road can increase drive.

6. **Create Measurable Goals:**
   - Make your goals measurable. Instead of saying "eat healthier," specify actions like "consume 20g of net carbs per day during the Induction Phase."

7. **Set a Timeline:**
   - Give each aim a reasonable timeline. This adds a sense of urgency and helps track progress effectively.

8. **Accountability:**
   - Talk to a friend, member of your family, or a support group about your objectives. Accountability can be a powerful motivator.

9. **Track Your Progress:**
   - Observe your development by keeping a journal. Record changes in weight, energy levels, and other relevant factors.

10. **Adaptability:**
    - Be willing to modify your objectives if necessary. Your priorities and circumstances may change, and your goals should reflect that flexibility.

11. **Celebrate Achievements:**

- Acknowledge and celebrate your successes. Whether big or small, recognizing achievements reinforces positive behavior.

Remember, setting and achieving goals is a dynamic process. Regularly reassess your objectives, make adjustments as needed, and celebrate the progress you've made on your Atkins Diet journey.

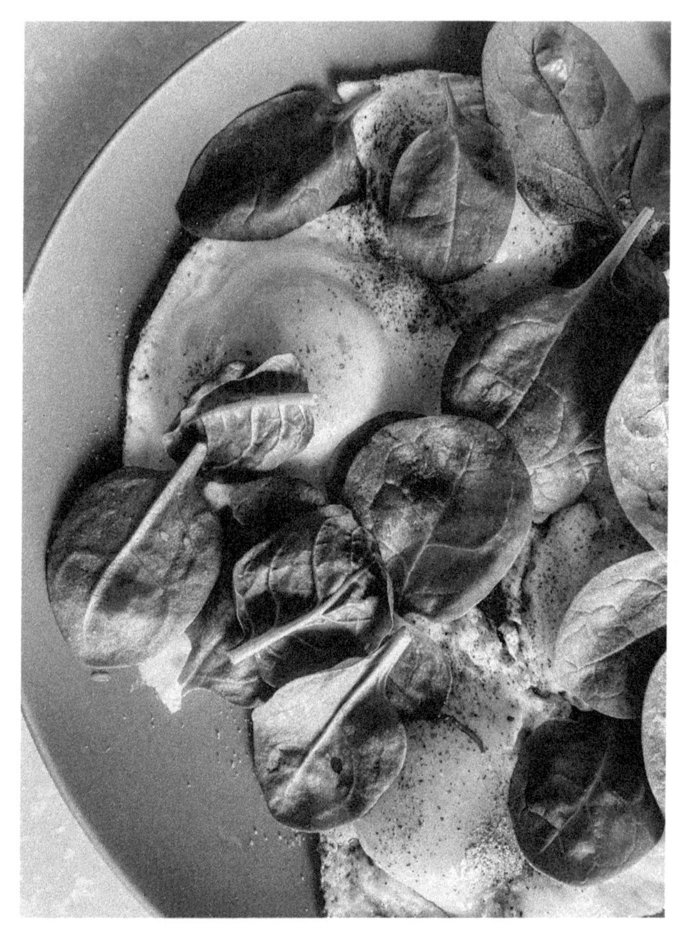

CHAPTER TWO

PHASE 1: INDUCTION

Phase 1 of the Atkins Diet is known as the "Induction Phase." This initial phase is crucial for kickstarting weight loss by transitioning the body into a state of ketosis. Here's an overview of Phase 1:

Objective:
- **Initiate Ketosis:** The primary goal of the Induction Phase is to restrict carbohydrate intake severely, typically to 20-25 grams of net carbs per day. This restriction prompts the body to enter ketosis, a metabolic state where it starts burning stored fat for energy.

Duration:
- **Typically 2 Weeks:** While the standard duration is two weeks, some individuals may choose to extend this phase based on their goals and how their body responds.

Carbohydrate Intake:
- **20-25 grams of Net Carbs:** Carbohydrates primarily come from low-carb vegetables. Fiber from these vegetables is subtracted from the total carb count to calculate net carbs.

Allowed Foods:

- **High-Fat, Moderate-Protein Foods:** Emphasis on animal proteins, eggs, and healthy fats such as olive oil and butter.
- **Low-Carb Vegetables:** Leafy greens, broccoli, cauliflower, and other non-starchy vegetables.

Restricted Foods:
- **High-Carb Foods:** Grains, fruits, legumes, and other high-carb options are restricted during this phase.

Beverages:
- **Water:** Hydration is crucial. Drink plenty of water throughout the day.
- **Herbal Tea and Coffee:** Unsweetened herbal tea and black coffee are typically allowed.

Supplements:
- **Multivitamin:** It's recommended to take a multivitamin to ensure you get essential nutrients during the carb-restricted phase.

Tips:
- **Monitor Ketosis:** Some individuals use ketone strips to monitor whether they have entered ketosis.
- **Portion Control:** Be mindful of portion sizes to manage caloric intake.
- **Listen to Your Body:** Pay attention to how your body responds and adjust your food choices accordingly.

The Induction Phase sets the foundation for the Atkins Diet and is designed to create a metabolic shift toward fat burning. Before beginning any large dietary changes, especially if you have underlying health conditions, it is crucial to speak with a healthcare provider.

INDUCTION GUIDELINES

The Induction Phase of the Atkins Diet comes with specific guidelines to help you successfully transition into ketosis and kickstart weight loss. Here are the key guidelines for the Induction Phase:

1. **Carbohydrate Intake:**
   - **Limit to 20-25 grams of Net Carbs:** Keep your daily carbohydrate intake within this range. Dietary fiber is deducted from total carbohydrates to determine net carbohydrates.

2. **Focus on Protein:**
   - **Moderate Protein Intake:** Include moderate amounts of protein in each meal to support muscle maintenance and satiety.

3. **Healthy Fats:**
   - **Emphasize Healthy Fats:** Incorporate healthy fats like olive oil, avocado, and butter to increase calorie intake and promote a feeling of fullness.

4. **Low-Carb Vegetables:**
   - **Include Non-Starchy Vegetables:** Prioritize vegetables with low carbohydrate content, such as leafy greens, broccoli, cauliflower, and spinach.

5. **Avoid High-Carb Foods:**
   - **Eliminate Grains, Fruits, and Legumes:** Restrict high-carb foods during this phase. This includes grains, fruits, and legumes.

6. **Beverages:**
   - **Hydration is Key:** Stay hydrated and promote general health throughout the day by sipping lots of water.
   - **Limit Caffeine Intake:** While some caffeine is allowed, excessive consumption may affect blood sugar levels for some individuals.

7. **Limit Dairy:**
   - **Moderate Dairy Intake:** Choose full-fat dairy products in moderation. Some individuals may be sensitive to dairy, so monitor how your body responds.

8. **Avoid Processed Foods:**
   - **Minimize Processed Foods:** Stick to whole, unprocessed foods to ensure you're not consuming hidden sugars or additives.

9. **Portion Control:**

   - **Be Mindful of Portions:** Pay attention to portion sizes to manage caloric intake. Overeating, even on low-carb foods, can hinder weight loss.

10. **Check Food Labels:**
   - **Read Labels Carefully:** Be diligent about checking food labels for hidden sugars and carbohydrate content.

11. **Track Progress:**
   - **Keep a Food Journal:** Record your daily food intake and monitor how your body responds to different foods.

12. **Listen to Your Body:**
   - **Be Attuned to Hunger and Fullness:** Eat when you're hungry and stop when you're satisfied. Pay attention to your body's signals.

Remember, individual responses to the Induction Phase may vary, and it's essential to listen to your body throughout the process. Consult with a healthcare professional before starting any significant dietary changes, especially if you have underlying health conditions.

Certainly! Here are three sample meal plans for the Induction Phase of the Atkins Diet, each with recipes and instructions:

Day 1:

Breakfast: Scrambled Eggs with Spinach and Feta
- **Ingredients:**
  - 3 eggs
  - Handful of fresh spinach
  - 2 tbsp feta cheese
  - Salt and pepper to taste
  - Butter for cooking
- **Instructions:**
  1. Beat the eggs and add salt and pepper to taste in a bowl.
  2. In a pan, melt butter over medium heat.
  3. Add spinach to the pan and cook until wilted.
  4. Pour beaten eggs over the spinach, add feta cheese, and scramble until cooked.

Lunch: Grilled Chicken Caesar Salad
- **Ingredients:**
  - Grilled chicken breast
  - Romaine lettuce
  - Cherry tomatoes
  - Parmesan cheese
  - Low-carb Caesar dressing

- **Instructions:**
   1. Grill chicken until fully cooked.
   2. Chop romaine lettuce, halve cherry tomatoes,
and shred Parmesan cheese.
   3. Slice grilled chicken and toss all ingredients
together. Drizzle with low-carb Caesar dressing.

Dinner: Baked Salmon with Lemon and Dill
- **Ingredients:**
   - Salmon fillets
   - Lemon slices
   - Fresh dill
   - Olive oil
- **Instructions:**
   1. Preheat oven to 375°F (190°C).
   2. Salmon fillets should be put on a baking pan.
   3. Top with lemon slices and fresh dill.
   4. Drizzle with olive oil and bake for 15-20 minutes
or until salmon is cooked through.

Day 2:

Breakfast: Vegetable Omelette
- **Ingredients:**
   - 3 eggs
   - Mushrooms
   - Bell peppers
   - Cheddar cheese
   - Olive oil
- **Instructions:**
   1. Beat eggs in a bowl and season with salt and
pepper.

2. In a pan, sauté mushrooms and bell peppers in olive oil.

3. Pour beaten eggs over vegetables and sprinkle cheddar cheese. Cook until eggs are set.

Lunch: Turkey and Avocado Lettuce Wraps
- **Ingredients:**
  - Sliced turkey
  - Lettuce leaves
  - Avocado slices
  - Mayonnaise
- **Instructions:**
  1. Lay out lettuce leaves.
  2. Add turkey slices and avocado.
  3. Drizzle with mayonnaise, roll up, and secure with toothpicks.

Dinner: Zucchini Noodles with Pesto and Shrimp
- **Ingredients:**
  - Zucchini noodles
  - Basil pesto made at home with pine nuts, garlic, basil, and olive oil
  - Grilled shrimp
- **Instructions:**
  1. Spiralize zucchini into noodles.
  2. In a pan, sauté zucchini noodles in pesto until tender.
  3. Top with grilled shrimp.

Day 3:

Breakfast: Greek Yogurt with Raspberries
- **Ingredients:**
  - Unsweetened, full-fat Greek yogurt
  - Handful of raspberries
- **Instructions:**
  1. Pour the Greek yogurt into a mixing dish.
  2. Top with fresh raspberries.

Lunch: Cobb Salad
- **Ingredients:**
  - Grilled chicken
  - Bacon
  - Avocado
  - Blue cheese dressing
- **Instructions:**
  1. Chop grilled chicken, bacon, and avocado.
  2. Toss all ingredients together and drizzle with blue cheese dressing.

Dinner: Beef Stir-Fry with Vegetables
- **Ingredients:**
  - Beef strips
  - Broccoli
  - Bell peppers
  - Snap peas
  - Coconut oil
- **Instructions:**
  1. Stir-fry beef strips in coconut oil until browned.
  2. Add chopped broccoli, bell peppers, and snap peas. Cook until vegetables are tender.

Portion proportions should be adjusted to meet your specific needs and tastes. Remember to stay within the recommended net carb limit during the Induction Phase. Enjoy your meals!

RECIPES FOR INDUCTION PHASE

Certainly! Here are three recipes suitable for the Induction Phase of the Atkins Diet:

Recipe 1: Chicken Breast with Spinach and Feta Stuffing

Ingredients:
- 2 boneless, skinless chicken breasts
- 1 cup fresh spinach, chopped
- 1/4 cup feta cheese, crumbled
- 1 clove garlic, minced
- Salt and pepper to taste
- Olive oil for cooking

Instructions:
1. Preheat the oven to 375°F (190°C).
2. In a bowl, mix chopped spinach, feta cheese, minced garlic, salt, and pepper.
3. On each of the chicken breasts, cut a pocket.
4. Stuff the pockets with the spinach and feta mixture.
5. Sprinkle salt and pepper on the outside of the chicken breasts.
6. In an oven-safe skillet, heat olive oil over medium-high heat.

7. Sear the chicken breasts for 2-3 minutes on each side.
8. Transfer the skillet to the preheated oven and bake for 20-25 minutes or until chicken is cooked through.

Recipe 2: Cauliflower Mash

Ingredients:
- 1 head cauliflower, chopped into florets
- 2 cloves garlic, minced
- 2 tbsp butter
- Salt and pepper to taste
- Chopped chives for garnish (optional)

Instructions:
1. Steam or boil cauliflower until tender.
2. Drain cauliflower and transfer to a food processor.
3. Add minced garlic, butter, salt, and pepper.
4. Blend until smooth and creamy.
5. Garnish with chopped chives if desired.

Recipe 3: Grilled Shrimp and Avocado Salad

Ingredients:
- 1 lb shrimp, peeled and deveined
- 2 tbsp olive oil
- 1 tsp cumin
- Salt and pepper to taste
- Mixed salad greens
- 1 avocado, sliced

- Cherry tomatoes, halved

Instructions:
1. In a bowl, toss shrimp with olive oil, cumin, salt, and pepper.
2. Elevate a skillet or grill to a medium-high temperature.
3. Grill shrimp for 2-3 minutes per side or until opaque.
4. In a large salad bowl, combine mixed greens, sliced avocado, and cherry tomatoes.
5. Top the salad with grilled shrimp.
6. Drizzle with additional olive oil and season with salt and pepper to taste.

Feel free to adjust these recipes based on your preferences, and enjoy these delicious and Atkins-friendly meals during the Induction Phase!

CHAPTER THREE

PHASE 2: BALANCING

Phase 2 of the Atkins Diet is known as the "Balancing Phase." This phase is designed to continue weight loss while gradually reintroducing more carbohydrates into your diet. Here's an overview of Phase 2:

Objectives:

1. **Gradual Carb Increase:**
   - Begin to increase your daily net carb intake by 5 grams each week.

2. **Monitor Individual Tolerance:**
   - Pay attention to how your body responds to the reintroduction of carbs. This helps determine your personal carb tolerance level.

3. **Continue Weight Loss:**
   - Aim to continue losing weight at a steady and sustainable pace.

Guidelines:

1. **Weekly Net Carb Increase:**
   - Increase net carbs by 5 grams each week until weight loss slows or stalls.

2. **Add More Vegetables:**
   - Include a variety of vegetables with slightly higher carb content, such as tomatoes, bell peppers, and onions.

3. **Introduce Nuts and Seeds:**
   - Gradually add nuts and seeds to your diet for additional nutrients and healthy fats.

4. **Explore Dairy Options:**
   - Introduce small amounts of dairy with higher carb content, such as yogurt or certain cheeses.

5. **Experiment with New Foods:**
   - Slowly introduce legumes and berries to your diet and monitor their impact on your weight loss progress.

6. **Stay Hydrated:**
   - Continue to prioritize water intake. Staying properly hydrated can help with weight loss and is important for general health.

Sample Meal Ideas:

1. **Grilled Chicken and Vegetable Skewers:**
   - Garlic, herbs, and olive oil are used to marinate chicken. Skewer with bell peppers, cherry tomatoes, and onions. Grill until chicken is cooked through.

2. **Salmon and Asparagus Bake:**

- Place salmon fillets and asparagus in a baking dish. Drizzle with olive oil and season with herbs. Bake until salmon flakes easily.

3. **Zoodle Stir-Fry with Shrimp:**
   - Stir-fry zucchini noodles with shrimp, broccoli, and snap peas in coconut oil and soy sauce.

4. **Cauliflower Rice Burrito Bowl:**
   - Top cauliflower rice with grilled chicken, salsa, guacamole, and a sprinkle of cheese.

5. **Greek Salad with Grilled Lamb:**
   - Mix together the cucumber, cherry tomatoes, feta cheese, olives, and mixed greens. Top with grilled lamb and a light olive oil dressing.

Remember to continue monitoring your progress and adjusting your carb intake based on your individual response. Gradually transitioning through the phases allows for a personalized and sustainable approach to the Atkins Diet. Seek the advice of a healthcare provider if you have any particular health concerns.

ADDING CARBS GRADUALLY

Gradually adding carbs is a key aspect of the Atkins Diet, especially during the Balancing Phase. Here's a step-by-step guide on how to add carbs gradually:

Week 1-2:

1. **Increase Net Carbs:**
   - Add 5 grams of net carbs per day. Focus on nutrient-dense vegetables with slightly higher carb content, like tomatoes and bell peppers.

2. **Sample Meals:**
   - Include a small serving of berries or half an apple with breakfast.
   - Add a side of roasted vegetables, such as sweet potatoes or carrots, to lunch or dinner.

3. **Monitor Response:**
   - Pay attention to your body's response. If weight loss continues and you feel good, you can maintain this level of carb intake.

Week 3-4:

1. **Additional Net Carb Increase:**
   - Add another 5 grams of net carbs per day, bringing your total increase to 10 grams. Consider introducing nuts and seeds.

2. **Sample Meals:**
   - Include a small handful of almonds or walnuts as a snack.
   - Add quinoa or brown rice as a side to a meal.

3. **Monitor Response:**

- Continue monitoring weight loss and how your body responds. Adjust the carb intake based on your progress.

Week 5-6:

1. **Further Increase in Net Carbs:**
   - Add another 5 grams of net carbs per day, reaching a total increase of 15 grams. Experiment with dairy options like yogurt or cheese.

2. **Sample Meals:**
   - Enjoy some Greek yogurt with berries on top.
   - Include a small portion of cheese with your meals.

3. **Monitor Response:**
   - Assess how your body reacts to the increased carb intake. Make adjustments as needed.

Week 7 Onward:

1. **Continue Gradual Increase:**
   - Continue adding 5 grams of net carbs per day every 1-2 weeks, focusing on a variety of whole foods.

2. **Explore Legumes and Whole Grains:**
   - Introduce legumes like lentils or chickpeas and experiment with whole grains like quinoa or barley.

3. **Individualize Your Diet:**

- Pay attention to your body's signals and individual tolerance. Your carb intake should be adjusted based on your weight loss goals and how your body responds.

Remember, the goal is to find the maximum amount of carbs you can consume while still losing or maintaining weight. This personalized approach ensures that you are in tune with your body and can sustain a healthy lifestyle. For individualized guidance, always speak with a medical professional or registered dietitian.

SAMPLE MEAL PLANS: BREAKFAST, LUNCH AND DINNER

Certainly! Here's a sample meal planning guide with a recipe for the Balancing Phase of the Atkins Diet. Let's focus on a day's worth of meals, including a delicious recipe for dinner:

Meal Planning Tips:

1. **Continue Gradual Carb Increase:**
   - Aim to increase net carbs by 5 grams per week during the Balancing Phase.

2. **Include a Variety of Vegetables:**
   - Incorporate a diverse range of low-carb vegetables, such as leafy greens, broccoli, cauliflower, bell peppers, and tomatoes.

3. **Experiment with Healthy Fats:**
   - Use healthy fats like olive oil, avocado oil, and butter in cooking. These fats contribute to satiety and flavor.

4. **Introduce Nuts and Seeds:**
   - Add nuts and seeds, such as almonds, walnuts, or chia seeds, as snacks or toppings to increase healthy fat and fiber intake.

5. **Include Lean Proteins:**
   - Choose lean protein sources like chicken, turkey, fish, and tofu to support muscle maintenance.

6. **Monitor Portion Sizes:**
   - Keep an eye on serving sizes to control your caloric consumption. Even with low-carb foods, overeating can hinder weight loss.

Sample Meal Plan:

Breakfast: Avocado and Spinach Omelette

Ingredients:
- 3 eggs
- 1/2 avocado, sliced
- Handful of fresh spinach
- Salt and pepper to taste
- Olive oil for cooking

Instructions:
1. Beat the eggs and add salt and pepper to taste in a bowl.
2. Heat olive oil in a pan over medium heat.
3. Add fresh spinach to the pan and cook until wilted.
4. Pour beaten eggs over the spinach, add sliced avocado, and cook until eggs are set.

Lunch: Grilled Chicken Salad with Roasted Vegetables

Ingredients:
- Grilled chicken breast, sliced
- Mixed salad greens
- Cherry tomatoes, halved
- Cucumber, sliced
- Red bell pepper, sliced
- Olive oil and balsamic vinegar dressing

Instructions:
1. Combine salad greens, cherry tomatoes, cucumber, and red bell pepper in a bowl.
2. Top with sliced grilled chicken.
3. Drizzle with olive oil and balsamic vinegar dressing.

Snack: Greek Yogurt with Berries

Ingredients:
- Unsweetened, full-fat Greek yogurt

- Mixed berries (strawberries, blueberries, raspberries)

Instructions:
1. Spoon Greek yogurt into a bowl.
2. Top with a mix of fresh berries.

Dinner: Lemon Garlic Butter Shrimp with Zucchini Noodles

Ingredients:
- 1 lb shrimp, peeled and deveined
- 3 medium-sized zucchini, spiralized
- 3 tbsp butter
- 3 cloves garlic, minced
- Juice of 1 lemon
- Salt and pepper to taste
- Fresh parsley for garnish

Instructions:
1. Add the butter to a pot and melt it over medium heat. Add the minced garlic and sauté it until fragrant.
2. Add shrimp to the pan and cook until opaque.
3. Add spiralized zucchini noodles to the pan and toss until just tender.
4. Squeeze lemon juice over the dish, season with salt and pepper, and garnish with fresh parsley.

Adapt serving sizes to your personal needs and degree of hunger. Remember to monitor your response to the gradual increase in net carbs and make adjustments accordingly. Enjoy your delicious and balanced meals!

DELICIOUS BALANCE RECIPES

Certainly! Here are three delicious recipes suitable for the Balancing Phase of the Atkins Diet:

Recipe 1: Grilled Chicken and Vegetable Skewers

Ingredients:
- Cut one pound of chicken breast into cubes
- Cherry tomatoes
- Bell peppers (assorted colors), cut into chunks
- Zucchini, sliced
- Red onion, cut into wedges
- Olive oil
- Add the paprika, salt, pepper, and garlic powder to taste.
- Wooden skewers, soaked in water

Instructions:
1. Preheat the grill or grill pan.
2. In a bowl, mix chicken cubes with olive oil, garlic powder, paprika, salt, and pepper.
3. Thread chicken, cherry tomatoes, bell peppers, zucchini, and red onion onto skewers.
4. Grill skewers until chicken is cooked through and vegetables are tender, turning occasionally.
5. Serve hot and enjoy!

Recipe 2: Salmon and Avocado Salad

Ingredients:
- 1 lb salmon fillets
- Mixed salad greens
- Avocado, sliced
- Cucumber, sliced
- Cherry tomatoes, halved
- Lemon vinaigrette (salt, pepper, Dijon mustard, lemon juice, and olive oil)

Instructions:
1. Use salt and pepper to season the salmon fillets.
2. Grill or bake salmon until flaky.
3. In a large bowl, combine salad greens, avocado, cucumber, and cherry tomatoes.
4. Top the salad with grilled salmon.
5. Drizzle with lemon vinaigrette before serving.

Recipe 3: Cauliflower and Broccoli Mash

Ingredients:
- 1 head cauliflower, chopped into florets
- 1 head broccoli, chopped into florets
- 2 cloves garlic, minced
- 2 tbsp butter
- Salt and pepper to taste
- Chopped chives for garnish

Instructions:
1. Steam or boil cauliflower and broccoli until tender.

2. Drain and transfer to a food processor.
3. Add minced garlic, butter, salt, and pepper.
4. Blend until smooth and creamy.
5. Garnish with chopped chives before serving.

You are welcome to modify these recipes to suit your dietary requirements and preferences. Incorporate a variety of colorful vegetables, lean proteins, and healthy fats to ensure a balanced and flavorful meal. Enjoy your delicious and nutritious meals during the Balancing Phase of the Atkins Diet!

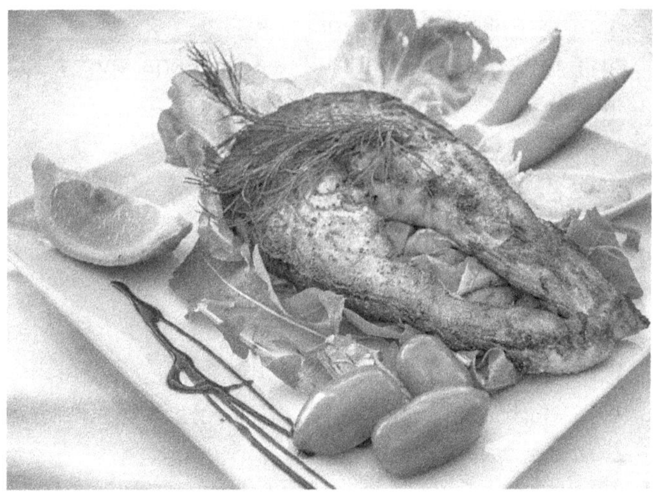

CHAPTER FOUR

PHASE 3: PRE-MAINTENANCE

Phase 3 of the Atkins Diet is known as "Pre-Maintenance." During this phase, you are approaching your weight loss goal, and the focus shifts to finding the right balance of carbohydrates that allows you to maintain your weight. Here's an overview:

Objectives:

1. **Fine-Tune Carb Intake:**
   - Continue increasing your daily net carb intake in 10-gram increments.

2. **Monitor Weight Loss:**
   - Aim for a slow and steady weight loss, transitioning towards weight maintenance.

3. **Discover Carb Tolerance:**
   - Identify your personal carbohydrate tolerance level by carefully introducing a wider variety of foods.

Guidelines:

1. **Weekly Net Carb Increase:**
   - Add 10 grams of net carbs per week to find your carbohydrate tolerance.

2. **Diversify Food Choices:**
   - Introduce a wider range of fruits, starchy vegetables, and whole grains.

3. **Evaluate Impact on Weight Loss:**
   - Monitor how each food group affects your weight. Adjust your carb intake based on your weight loss goals.

4. **Maintain Adequate Protein:**
   - Ensure you are getting enough protein to support muscle maintenance.

5. **Stay Hydrated:**
   - Continue prioritizing hydration. Water intake is crucial for overall health and weight management.

Sample Meal Ideas:

1. **Quinoa and Vegetable Stir-Fry:**
   - Stir-fry quinoa with a variety of colorful vegetables, tofu or lean protein, and a light soy sauce.

2. **Baked Sweet Potato with Grilled Chicken:**
   - Top a baked sweet potato with grilled chicken, Greek yogurt, and a sprinkle of chives.

3. **Mixed Berry Smoothie:**

- Blend mixed berries with unsweetened almond milk and a scoop of protein powder for a delicious smoothie.

4. **Whole Grain Wrap with Turkey and Avocado:**
   - Fill a whole grain wrap with sliced turkey, avocado, lettuce, and a dollop of Greek yogurt.

5. **Mango Salsa Tilapia:**
   - Bake tilapia fillets with a topping of mango salsa made with diced mango, tomatoes, onions, cilantro, and lime juice.

Tips for Success:

1. **Listen to Your Body:**
   - Keep an eye on how your body reacts to various foods. Note any changes in energy levels, cravings, or weight fluctuations.

2. **Regular Exercise:**
   - Incorporate regular physical activity to support overall health and weight maintenance.

3. **Regular Check-ins:**
   - Periodically reassess your weight loss goals and adjust your carbohydrate intake accordingly.

4. **Stay Informed:**
   - Stay informed about the nutritional content of foods to make informed choices.

5. **Seek Professional Guidance:**
   - Consult a qualified dietician or other healthcare professional for personalized advice.

Remember, the Pre-Maintenance Phase is a transition towards long-term weight maintenance. It's about figuring out a fun and sustainable eating pattern that suits your needs. Adjust your carbohydrate intake based on your individual needs and goals.

APPROACHING YOUR GOAL WEIGHT

Approaching your goal weight is an exciting phase, and it requires a thoughtful and sustainable approach to ensure you reach and maintain your desired weight. Here are some tips as you approach your goal weight:

1. **Fine-Tune Nutrition:**
   - Continue gradually increasing your net carb intake, monitoring its impact on your weight loss progress.
   - Focus on nutrient-dense foods, incorporating a variety of vegetables, lean proteins, and healthy fats.

2. **Monitor Portion Sizes:**
   - Pay attention to portion sizes to avoid overeating, even with low-carb foods.

3. **Diversify Food Choices:**
   - Introduce a wider range of foods, including fruits, starchy vegetables, and whole grains.
   - Try a variety of dishes to keep your meals fulfilling and engaging.

4. **Regular Exercise:**
   - Incorporate regular physical activity into your routine to support overall health and weight maintenance.

5. **Hydration is Key:**
   - Continue prioritizing hydration. Adequate water intake supports various bodily functions and can help manage hunger.

6. **Stay Mindful:**
   - Practice mindful eating. Be aware of hunger and fullness cues to avoid unnecessary snacking.

7. **Regular Check-ins:**
   - Evaluate your progress on a regular basis and modify your strategy as necessary. Consider keeping a food journal to track your meals and emotions.

8. **Celebrate Small Wins:**
   - Recognize and celebrate your advancements as you go. It's critical to acknowledge your diligence and hard work.

9. **Listen to Your Body:**
   - Pay attention to how your body responds to different meals and adjust your diet accordingly.
   - Be mindful of stress levels and ensure you're getting enough sleep.

10. **Seek Professional Guidance:**
   - Consult with a registered dietitian or healthcare professional for personalized advice and support.

11. **Set Realistic Goals:**
   - Establish realistic and achievable goals. This may involve adjusting your expectations as you get closer to your goal weight.

12. **Maintain a Balanced Lifestyle:**
   - Aim for a balanced and sustainable lifestyle that includes healthy eating, regular exercise, and adequate self-care.

13. **Reassess and Adapt:**
   - Be open to reassessing your approach and adapting to changes. Our bodies can change, as can our dietary needs.

14. **Enjoy the Journey:**
   - Embrace the journey and the positive changes you've made. Celebrate the improvements in your overall well-being.

Recall that maintaining a healthy weight requires sustained effort. Focus on building habits that contribute to your overall well-being, and enjoy the process of becoming the healthiest version of yourself.

INTRODUCTION OF MORE CARBS

Certainly! Here are three recipes to help you introduce more carbs gradually while maintaining a balanced approach. These recipes incorporate whole, unprocessed carbohydrates along with other nutrient-dense ingredients:

Recipe 1: Quinoa and Roasted Vegetable Bowl

Ingredients:
- 1 cup cooked quinoa
- Assorted vegetables (bell peppers, cherry tomatoes, zucchini, red onion), chopped
- Olive oil
- Garlic powder, cumin, paprika
- Salt and pepper to taste
- Feta cheese (optional)

Instructions:
1. Preheat the oven to 400°F (200°C).
2. Toss chopped vegetables in olive oil, garlic powder, cumin, paprika, salt, and pepper.
3. Roast the vegetables on a baking sheet for 20-25 minutes or until tender.
4. In a bowl, combine cooked quinoa and roasted vegetables.

5. Top with crumbled feta cheese if desired.

Recipe 2: Berry and Almond Yogurt Parfait

Ingredients:
- 1 cup Greek yogurt
- Mixed berries (strawberries, blueberries, raspberries)
- Almonds, chopped
- Honey (optional)
- Granola (optional)

Instructions:
1. Arrange Greek yogurt layers in a glass or bowl.
2. Add a layer of mixed berries and chopped almonds.
3. Repeat the layers.
4. Drizzle with honey and sprinkle granola on top if desired.

Recipe 3: Sweet Potato and Chickpea Buddha Bowl

Ingredients:
- 1 medium sweet potato, diced
- 1 can chickpeas, drained and rinsed
- Olive oil
- Cumin, smoked paprika, garlic powder
- Salt and pepper to taste
- Baby spinach
- Avocado, sliced
- Tahini dressing

Instructions:
1. Preheat the oven to 425°F (220°C).
2. Toss diced sweet potato and chickpeas in olive oil, cumin, smoked paprika, garlic powder, salt, and pepper.
3. Roast in the oven for 25-30 minutes or until sweet potatoes are tender.
4. Assemble bowls with a base of baby spinach, roasted sweet potatoes, chickpeas, and sliced avocado.
5. Drizzle with tahini dressing before serving.

Instructions for the Transition Period:

1. **Portion Control:**
   - Start with smaller portions of these carb-rich recipes and monitor your body's response.

2. **Observe Energy Levels:**
   - Pay attention to how your body reacts to the increased carb intake. Adjust portions or types of carbs if needed.

3. **Track Progress:**
   - Keep a food diary to track your meals, energy levels, and any changes in weight.

4. **Personalize:**
   - Adjust ingredients or quantities based on your individual preferences and nutritional needs.

Remember to enjoy the process of experimenting with new foods and finding the balance that works best for you during this transition. Adjustments can be made based on your body's response and your overall health goals.

PRE-MAINTENANCE RECIPES

Certainly! Here are three delicious and nutritious recipes suitable for the Pre-Maintenance phase of the Atkins Diet:

Recipe 1: Mediterranean Quinoa Bowl

Ingredients:
- 1 cup cooked quinoa
- Grilled chicken breast, sliced
- Cherry tomatoes, halved
- Cucumber, diced
- Kalamata olives, sliced
- Red onion, finely chopped
- Feta cheese, crumbled
- Fresh parsley, chopped
- Olive oil and lemon juice
- Salt and pepper to taste

Instructions:
1. In a large bowl, combine cooked quinoa, grilled chicken, cherry tomatoes, cucumber, Kalamata olives, red onion, and feta cheese.
2. Drizzle olive oil and lemon juice over the bowl.
3. Toss gently to combine.

4. To taste, add salt and pepper for seasoning.
5. Garnish with fresh parsley before serving.

Recipe 2: Shrimp and Avocado Salad

Ingredients:
- 1 lb shrimp, peeled and deveined
- Mixed salad greens
- Avocado, sliced
- Cherry tomatoes, halved
- Red bell pepper, sliced
- Cilantro, chopped
- Lime vinaigrette (lime juice, olive oil, garlic, salt, and pepper)

Instructions:
1. In a pan, cook shrimp until opaque and cooked through.
2. In a large bowl, combine mixed salad greens, avocado, cherry tomatoes, red bell pepper, and cooked shrimp.
3. In a small bowl, whisk together lime juice, olive oil, minced garlic, salt, and pepper to make the vinaigrette.
4. Pour the vinaigrette onto the salad and give it a little stir.
5. Garnish with chopped cilantro before serving.

Recipe 3: Quinoa Stuffed Bell Peppers

Ingredients:
- Bell peppers, halved and seeds removed

- 1 cup cooked quinoa
- Ground turkey or lean ground beef
- Onion, diced
- Black beans, drained and rinsed
- Corn kernels
- Taco seasoning
- Shredded cheese
- Fresh cilantro, chopped

Instructions:
1. Preheat the oven to 375°F (190°C).
2. In a pan, cook ground turkey or beef with diced onion until browned.
3. Add taco seasoning, black beans, corn, and cooked quinoa to the pan. Mix well.
4. Stuff bell pepper halves with the quinoa and meat mixture.
5. Top with shredded cheese.
6. Bake in the oven for 20-25 minutes or until peppers are tender.
7. Garnish with chopped cilantro before serving.

Instructions for the Pre-Maintenance Phase:

1. **Portion Control:**
   - Pay attention to portion sizes and adjust based on your energy needs and weight management goals.

2. **Monitor Energy Levels:**
   - Observe how your body responds to the increased carb intake. Adjust quantities if needed.

3. **Personalize Recipes:**
   - Customize these recipes to suit your taste preferences and nutritional requirements.

4. **Enjoy Variety:**
   - Explore a diverse range of ingredients to keep your meals interesting and satisfying.

5. **Stay Hydrated:**
   - Continue prioritizing hydration as you introduce more carbs into your diet.

Feel free to adapt these recipes based on your preferences, and remember to embrace the variety of flavors and nutrients that a balanced diet offers during the Pre-Maintenance phase.

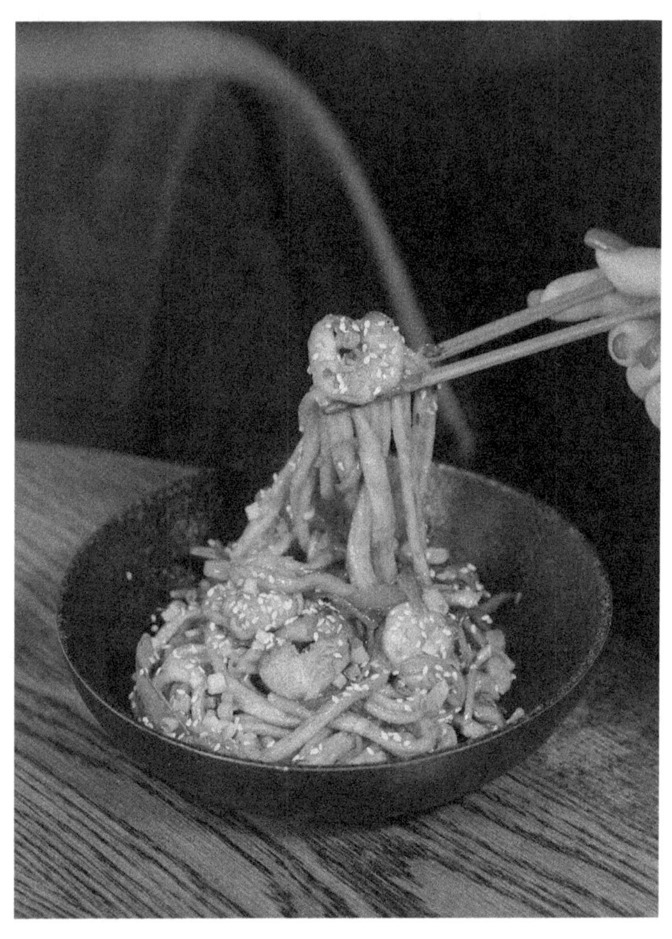

CHAPTER FIVE

PHASE 4: MAINTENANCE

Congratulations on reaching the Maintenance Phase of the Atkins Diet! This phase is about sustaining the healthy habits you've developed and maintaining your weight loss. Here's an overview:

Objectives:

1. **Stabilize Weight:**
   - Maintain your achieved weight loss goal.

2. **Establish Long-Term Habits:**
   - Solidify the healthy eating habits and lifestyle changes you've adopted during the previous phases.

3. **Flexible Carb Intake:**
   - Enjoy a flexible approach to carb intake, finding the balance that works best for your body.

Guidelines:

1. **Monitor Weight Regularly:**
   - Regularly weigh yourself to ensure you stay within your target weight range.

2. **Flexible Carb Range:**

- Find your personal carb tolerance level. Some may comfortably consume a higher carb count, while others may prefer a more moderate approach.

3. **Healthy Lifestyle Habits:**
   - Continue incorporating regular physical activity, staying hydrated, and practicing mindful eating.

4. **Balance Macronutrients:**
   - Maintain a balance between carbohydrates, proteins, and fats for overall health.

5. **Listen to Your Body:**
   - Pay attention to your body's signals. Adjust your diet based on energy levels, cravings, and overall well-being.

6. **Celebrate Success:**
   - Acknowledge and celebrate your achievements. Think back on the improvements you've achieved.

Sample Meal Ideas:

1. **Grilled Salmon with Asparagus and Quinoa:**
   - Grilled salmon served with asparagus and a side of quinoa.

2. **Mediterranean Chicken Salad:**
   - Grilled chicken breast over a bed of mixed greens, cherry tomatoes, cucumber, olives, and feta cheese, dressed with olive oil and lemon juice.

3. **Vegetarian Stir-Fry:**
   - Colorful stir-fried vegetables (bell peppers, broccoli, snap peas) with tofu, served over cauliflower rice.

4. **Turkey and Avocado Lettuce Wraps:**
   - Ground turkey cooked with spices, wrapped in lettuce leaves with sliced avocado.

5. **Berry and Almond Yogurt Parfait:**
   - Greek yogurt layered with mixed berries, chopped almonds, and a drizzle of honey.

Tips for Success:

1. **Regular Check-ins:**
   - Periodically reassess your weight and adjust your carb intake accordingly.

2. **Lifestyle Balance:**
   - Ensure a balanced lifestyle that includes not only healthy eating but also regular exercise, quality sleep, and stress management.

3. **Adapt to Changes:**
   - Be open to adjusting your approach based on changes in your activity level, lifestyle, or health status.

4. **Seek Professional Guidance:**

- Consult with a registered dietitian or healthcare professional for ongoing support and personalized advice.

Remember, the Maintenance Phase is about finding a sustainable and enjoyable way of eating that supports both your weight maintenance goals and overall well-being. Continue to make informed choices and embrace the lifestyle that aligns with your health objectives.

MAINTAINING WEIGHT LOSS

Maintaining weight loss is a long-term commitment that involves sustaining healthy habits and making lifestyle adjustments. Here are some key tips to help you maintain your weight loss:

1. **Stay Active:**
   - Continue incorporating regular physical activity into your routine. Make an effort to include cardiovascular exercise, strength training, and flexibility training in your regimen.

2. **Balanced Nutrition:**
   - Maintain a balanced diet with a variety of nutrient-dense foods. Give priority to entire grains, fruits, vegetables, lean meats, and healthy fats.

3. **Portion Control:**

- Be mindful of portion sizes. To avoid overindulging, pay attention to your body's cues of hunger and fullness.

4. **Regular Monitoring:**
   - Periodically monitor your weight to catch any changes early. Regular check-ins can help you make timely adjustments.

5. **Flexible Carb Intake:**
   - Embrace a flexible approach to carbohydrate intake. Find the level that supports your energy needs while maintaining weight.

6. **Hydration:**
   - Throughout the day, consume plenty of water to stay hydrated. Feelings of hunger can occasionally be confused with dehydration.

7. **Mindful Eating:**
   - Practice mindful eating by savoring your meals, eating slowly, and paying attention to hunger and fullness cues.

8. **Regular Sleep:**
   - Prioritize quality sleep as it plays a crucial role in overall health and weight management.

9. **Manage Stress:**
   - Use stress-reduction strategies including yoga, meditation, and deep breathing exercises.

10. **Healthy Habits:**
   - Continue with the healthy habits you developed during your weight loss journey, including regular exercise, nutritious eating, and positive lifestyle choices.

11. **Social Support:**
   - Surround yourself with a supportive network of friends, family, or a weight loss community. Talk about your experiences and ask for help when you need it.

12. **Adaptability:**
   - Be adaptable to changes in your life, such as schedule adjustments, travel, or special occasions. Plan ahead to make healthier choices during such times.

13. **Celebrate Achievements:**
   - Recognize and celebrate your advancements as you go. Acknowledge the gains and constructive adjustments you've made.

14. **Professional Guidance:**
   - Seek advice from a qualified dietician or other healthcare provider if necessary. They can provide specialized advice and support.

15. **Lifelong Mindset:**
   - Adopt a mindset that recognizes maintaining a healthy weight is a lifelong journey. Embrace the positive impact on your overall well-being.

Remember, maintaining weight loss is about finding a sustainable and enjoyable lifestyle that aligns with your health goals. It's not just about reaching a number on the scale but fostering habits that contribute to your overall well-being.

SUSTAINABLE EATING HABIT

Sustainable eating habits are key to long-term health and well-being. Here are principles to guide you in adopting sustainable eating habits:

1. **Balanced and Varied Diet:**
   - Aim for a balanced mix of fruits, vegetables, whole grains, lean proteins, and healthy fats to ensure you receive a broad range of nutrients.

2. **Portion Control:**
   - Be mindful of portion sizes to avoid overindulging. Listen to your body's hunger and fullness cues.

3. **Whole, Unprocessed Foods:**
   - Give complete, raw meals precedence over heavily processed ones. Choose foods in their natural state for optimal nutritional value.

4. **Hydration:**

- Stay hydrated by sipping plenty of water throughout the day. Choose water, herbal teas, or infused water instead of sugar-filled beverages.

5. **Mindful Eating:**
   - Savor each bite, eat carefully, and pay attention to your body's hunger and fullness cues as you practice mindful eating.

6. **Meal Planning:**
   - Plan your meals ahead of time to make informed choices and avoid impulsive, less nutritious options.

7. **Incorporate Variety:**
   - Include a variety of foods in your diet to ensure a diverse range of nutrients. Experiment with new recipes and cuisines.

8. **Flexibility:**
   - Be flexible in your eating approach. Allow yourself occasional treats without guilt, focusing on overall balance.

9. **Local and Seasonal Produce:**
   - Whenever possible, choose locally sourced and seasonal produce. It's often fresher, supports local farmers, and has a lower environmental impact.

10. **Mindful Food Sourcing:**

- Consider the environmental and ethical impact of your food choices. Choose sustainably sourced and ethically produced foods.

11. **Limit Added Sugars and Salt:**
   - Minimize the intake of added sugars and excessive salt. Check food labels and choose options with lower added sugars and sodium content.

12. **Cook at Home:**
   - When you create meals at home, you have complete control over the ingredients and cooking processes. It's often more cost-effective and healthier.

13. **Regular Physical Activity:**
   - Combine healthy eating with regular physical activity to promote overall well-being.

14. **Social Connection:**
   - Enjoy meals with friends and family. Social connections during meals can contribute to a positive and satisfying eating experience.

15. **Educate Yourself:**
   - Stay informed about nutritional content, food labeling, and the impact of your food choices on your health and the environment.

16. **Set Realistic Goals:**

- Establish achievable and realistic goals. Small, consistent changes over time are more likely to lead to sustainable habits.

17. **Professional Guidance:**
   - Consult with a registered dietitian or nutritionist for personalized advice and support tailored to your specific needs.

By adopting these sustainable eating habits, you can create a foundation for a healthier and more balanced lifestyle that you can maintain in the long run.

MAINTENANCE-FRIENDLY RECIPES

Certainly! Here are three maintenance-friendly recipes that focus on balanced nutrition and are suitable for maintaining a healthy weight:

Recipe 1: Grilled Chicken and Quinoa Salad

Ingredients:
- Grilled chicken breast, sliced
- 1 cup cooked quinoa
- Mixed salad greens
- Cherry tomatoes, halved
- Cucumber, sliced
- Red onion, thinly sliced
- Feta cheese, crumbled
- Olive oil and balsamic vinegar
- Salt and pepper to taste

Instructions:
1. In a large bowl, combine grilled chicken, cooked quinoa, mixed salad greens, cherry tomatoes, cucumber, red onion, and feta cheese.
2. Pour over some olive oil and balsamic vinegar.
3. Toss gently to combine.
4. To taste, add salt and pepper for seasoning.
5. Serve chilled or at room temperature.

Recipe 2: Salmon and Vegetable Stir-Fry

Ingredients:
- One-pound salmon fillets, sliced into pieces
- Broccoli florets
- Bell peppers, sliced
- Snap peas
- Carrots, julienned
- Garlic, minced
- Ginger, grated
- Low-sodium soy sauce
- Sesame oil
- Brown rice, cooked

Instructions:
1. In a wok or large skillet, heat sesame oil over medium-high heat.
2. Add salmon chunks and stir-fry until cooked.
3. Add garlic and ginger, stir-frying for a minute.
4. Add broccoli, bell peppers, snap peas, and carrots. Stir-fry until vegetables are tender-crisp.
5. Pour in low-sodium soy sauce and toss to coat.

6. Serve over cooked brown rice.

Recipe 3: Greek Yogurt Parfait with Berries and Almonds

Ingredients:
- Greek yogurt
- Mixed berries (strawberries, blueberries, raspberries)
- Almonds, sliced
- Honey or maple syrup
- Granola (optional)

Instructions:
1. Arrange Greek yogurt layers in a glass or bowl.
2. Add a layer of mixed berries and sliced almonds.
3. Repeat the layers.
4. Drizzle with honey or maple syrup.
5. Optionally, sprinkle granola on top for added crunch.

Tips for Maintenance-Friendly Eating:

1. **Portion Awareness:**
   - Be mindful of portion sizes to support weight maintenance.

2. **Balance Macros:**
   - Every meal should contain a variety of healthful fats, carbs, and proteins.

3. **Whole Foods:**

   - Give whole, high-nutrient foods precedence over processed ones.

4. **Hydration:**
   - Stay well-hydrated throughout the day.

5. **Flexibility:**
   - Allow flexibility in your diet to enjoy a variety of foods in moderation.

6. **Listen to Your Body:**
   - Observe your body's signals of hunger and fullness.

7. **Regular Physical Activity:**
   - Keep adding regular exercise to your daily regimen.

Remember to customize these recipes based on your preferences and dietary needs. Enjoy the delicious flavors while maintaining a healthy and balanced lifestyle.

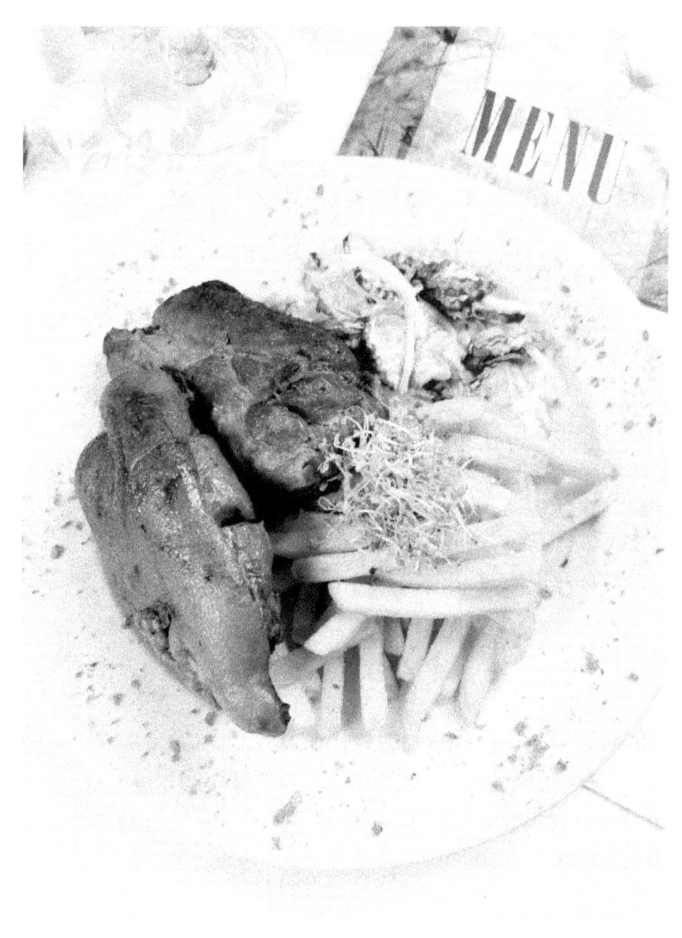
MENU

CHAPTER SIX

SNACKS AND QUICK MEALS

Certainly! Here are three quick and nutritious snack ideas, along with three easy-to-make quick meals for a satisfying and balanced approach:

Snack Ideas:

1. Greek Yogurt and Berry Bowl:
- Greek yogurt
- Mixed berries (strawberries, blueberries, raspberries)
- Almonds, chopped
- Honey or maple syrup

Instructions:
1. In a bowl, combine Greek yogurt with mixed berries.
2. Sprinkle chopped almonds on top.
3. For sweetness, drizzle with maple syrup or honey.

2. Hummus and Veggie Sticks:
- Hummus
- Carrot sticks
- Cucumber slices
- Cherry tomatoes

Instructions:

1. Dip carrot sticks, cucumber slices, and cherry tomatoes in hummus.
2. Enjoy a crunchy and satisfying snack.

3. Nut Butter Banana Bites:
- Banana, sliced
- Nut butter (almond, peanut, or any preferred)
- Chia seeds (optional)

Instructions:
1. Spread nut butter on banana slices.
2. Sprinkle chia seeds on top for added texture.
3. Arrange on a plate and enjoy.

Quick Meal Ideas:

1. Quinoa and Vegetable Stir-Fry:
- Cooked quinoa
- Mixed vegetables (bell peppers, broccoli, snap peas)
- Tofu or grilled chicken
- Soy sauce
- Sesame oil

Instructions:
1. Stir-fry mixed vegetables in sesame oil.
2. Add cooked quinoa and protein of choice.
3. Drizzle with soy sauce and toss until well combined.

2. Caprese Salad with Avocado:
- Cherry tomatoes, halved

- Fresh mozzarella, sliced
- Avocado, diced
- Fresh basil leaves
- Balsamic glaze
- Olive oil

Instructions:
1. Arrange cherry tomatoes, mozzarella, and avocado on a plate.
2. Garnish with fresh basil leaves.
3. Pour balsamic glaze and olive oil over.

3. Turkey and Veggie Wrap:
- Whole grain wrap
- Turkey slices
- Hummus
- Spinach leaves
- Sliced bell peppers
- Cherry tomatoes, halved

Instructions:
1. Spread hummus on a whole grain wrap.
2. Layer with turkey slices, spinach leaves, bell peppers, and cherry tomatoes.
3. Roll up and secure with toothpicks.

Tips for Quick Meals and Snacks:

1. **Prep Ahead:**
   - Keep pre-cut veggies, cooked quinoa, or grilled chicken in the fridge for quick assembly.

2. **Smart Substitutions:**
   - Experiment with ingredient substitutions based on your preferences and dietary needs.

3. **Batch Cooking:**
   - Prepare larger quantities of grains, proteins, and veggies during meal prep to use in multiple meals.

4. **Portion Control:**
   - Pay attention to portion sizes to maintain balance in your quick meals and snacks.

5. **Hydration:**
   - Make sure you stay hydrated throughout the day by sipping herbal tea or water.

These snack and meal ideas are versatile, allowing you to customize them based on your taste and dietary preferences. Enjoy the convenience of quick, nutritious options to keep you fueled and satisfied!

LOW-CARB SNACK IDEAS

Certainly! Here are five low-carb snack ideas that are both delicious and satisfying:

1. **Cheese and Pepperoni Bites:**
   - Cheese cubes (cheddar, mozzarella, or your favorite cheese)
   - Pepperoni slices

Instructions:
   1. Alternate threading cheese cubes and
pepperoni slices onto toothpicks.
   2. Enjoy this savory and protein-rich snack.

2. **Cucumber and Cream Cheese Roll-Ups:**
   - Cucumber slices
   - Cream cheese
   - Smoked salmon or turkey slices

Instructions:
   1. Spread a thin layer of cream cheese on
cucumber slices.
   2. Place a small piece of smoked salmon or
turkey on each slice.
   3. Roll them up for a refreshing and low-carb
snack.

3. **Avocado and Tuna Salad:**
   - Avocado, diced
   - Canned tuna, drained
   - Lemon juice
   - Salt and pepper to taste

Instructions:
   1. In a bowl, mix diced avocado and canned tuna.
   2. Drizzle with lemon juice and season with salt
and pepper.

4. **Hard-Boiled Eggs with Guacamole:**
   - Hard-boiled eggs, sliced

- Guacamole

Instructions:
   1. Slice hard-boiled eggs and serve with a side of guacamole.
   2. This combination provides healthy fats and protein.

5. **Zucchini Noodles with Pesto:**
   - Zucchini noodles (zoodles)
   - Pesto sauce
   - Cherry tomatoes, halved

Instructions:
   1. Toss zucchini noodles with pesto sauce.
   2. Add halved cherry tomatoes for a low-carb and flavorful snack.

Tips for Low-Carb Snacking:

1. **Portion Control:**
   - Be mindful of portion sizes to maintain a balance of nutrients.

2. **Hydration:**
   - To stay hydrated, pair your snacks with water or herbal tea.

3. **Nuts and Seeds:**
   - Enjoy a handful of nuts or seeds for a crunchy and satisfying option.

4. **Vegetable Sticks with Dip:**
   - Dip celery, cucumber, or bell pepper strips into guacamole or a low-carb dip.

5. **Berries with Whipped Cream:**
   - Indulge in a small portion of berries topped with unsweetened whipped cream for a sweet treat.

Remember to personalize these snacks based on your preferences and dietary requirements. These low-carb options provide a mix of healthy fats and protein to keep you energized throughout the day.

QUICK AND EASY RECIPES FOR BUSY DAYS

Absolutely! Here are three quick and easy recipes perfect for busy days:

Recipe 1: One-Pan Chicken and Vegetables

Ingredients:
- Chicken breast or thighs, boneless and skinless
- Various veggies, including cherry tomatoes, bell peppers, and broccoli
- Olive oil
- Garlic powder
- Paprika
- Salt and pepper

Instructions:

1. Preheat the oven to 400°F (200°C).
2. Place chicken and vegetables on a baking sheet.
3. Drizzle with olive oil and sprinkle with garlic powder, paprika, salt, and pepper.
4. Toss everything to coat evenly.
5. Bake the chicken for 20 to 25 minutes, or until it is thoroughly done.

Recipe 2: Quick Shrimp Stir-Fry

Ingredients:
- Shrimp, peeled and deveined
- Mixed vegetables stir-fried (carrots, broccoli, and snap peas)
- Soy sauce
- Sesame oil
- Garlic, minced
- Ginger, grated
- Cooked rice or cauliflower rice

Instructions:
1. In a wok or skillet, heat sesame oil over medium-high heat.
2. Add shrimp, garlic, and ginger. Cook until shrimp turn pink.
3. Add stir-fry vegetables and cook until they're tender-crisp.
4. Drizzle with soy sauce and toss everything together.
5. Serve over cooked rice or cauliflower rice.

Recipe 3: Avocado and Chickpea Salad

Ingredients:
- Canned chickpeas, drained and rinsed
- Avocado, diced
- Cherry tomatoes, halved
- Red onion, finely chopped
- Cilantro, chopped
- Olive oil
- Lemon juice
- Salt and pepper

Instructions:
1. In a bowl, combine chickpeas, avocado, cherry tomatoes, red onion, and cilantro.
2. Pour in some lemon juice and olive oil.
3. Season with salt and pepper.
4. Toss gently to combine, and your salad is ready.

Tips for Quick Cooking on Busy Days:

1. **Prep Ingredients in Advance:**
   - Chop vegetables or marinate proteins ahead of time.

2. **Use Convenient Cooking Methods:**
   - Opt for one-pan dishes, stir-fries, or sheet pan meals for easy cleanup.

3. **Keep Staple Ingredients Handy:**
   - Have pantry staples like canned beans, rice, and frozen vegetables for quick assembly.

4. **Utilize Quick Proteins:**
   - Choose fast-cooking proteins like shrimp or thinly sliced chicken.

5. **Batch Cooking:**
   - Prepare larger quantities and refrigerate or freeze for future quick meals.

6. **Simple Seasonings:**
   - Use versatile seasonings like garlic powder, paprika, and soy sauce for added flavor.

7. **Shortcut Ingredients:**
   - Utilize pre-cut veggies, pre-cooked grains, or pre-marinated proteins for time-saving.

Remember to adapt these recipes based on your taste preferences and dietary needs. Quick and easy doesn't mean sacrificing flavor or nutrition!

CHAPTER SEVEN

DESSERTS AND TREATS

Certainly! Here are three delightful dessert and treat ideas that are not only delicious but also relatively quick to prepare:

Recipe 1: Chia Seed Pudding with Berries

Ingredients:
- 1/4 cup chia seeds
- One cup almond milk (or your favorite type of milk)
- 1-2 tablespoons maple syrup or honey
- 1/2 teaspoon vanilla extract
- Mixed berries (strawberries, blueberries, raspberries)

Instructions:
1. In a bowl, whisk together chia seeds, almond milk, maple syrup (or honey), and vanilla extract.
2. Let the mixture sit for 10 minutes, then stir again to prevent clumping.
3. Refrigerate for at least 2 hours or overnight.
4. Before serving, layer the chia pudding with mixed berries.
5. Optional: Add a drizzle of extra maple syrup or honey on top.

Recipe 2: Dark Chocolate Avocado Mousse

Ingredients:
- 2 ripe avocados
- 1/4 cup cocoa powder
- One-fourth cup of pure agave or pure maple syrup
- 1/2 teaspoon vanilla extract
- A pinch of salt
- Dark chocolate shavings for garnish

Instructions:
1. In a blender or food processor, combine avocados, cocoa powder, maple syrup, vanilla extract, and salt.
2. Blend until smooth and creamy.
3. Spoon the mousse into serving bowls.
4. Place in the fridge to chill for a minimum of half an hour.
5. Garnish with dark chocolate shavings before serving.

Recipe 3: Almond Butter Energy Bites

Ingredients:
- 1 cup rolled oats
- 1/2 cup almond butter
- 1/3 cup honey or maple syrup
- 1/2 cup ground flaxseed
- 1/2 cup dark chocolate chips
- 1 teaspoon vanilla extract
- A pinch of salt

Instructions:

1. In a bowl, mix together rolled oats, almond
butter, honey (or maple syrup), ground flaxseed,
chocolate chips, vanilla extract, and salt.
2. Refrigerate the mixture for 15-30 minutes to
make it easier to handle.
3. Take small portions and roll into bite-sized balls.
4. Place the energy bites on a tray and refrigerate
for at least 1 hour before serving.

Tips for Healthier Desserts and Treats:

1. **Use Natural Sweeteners:**
   - Choose natural sweeteners such as agave
nectar, honey, or maple syrup.

2. **Incorporate Fruit:**
   - Include fresh fruits in your desserts for natural
sweetness.

3. **Choose Dark Chocolate:**
   - When using chocolate, choose dark chocolate
for a richer flavor and potential health benefits.

4. **Experiment with Nuts and Seeds:**
   - Add nuts or seeds for a satisfying crunch and
added nutritional value.

5. **Portion Control:**
   - Enjoy desserts in moderation to maintain a
balanced diet.

Feel free to customize these recipes to suit your taste preferences and dietary requirements. These treats are designed to bring joy without compromising on health-conscious choices.

LOW-CARB DESSERTS OPTIONS

Certainly! Here are three low-carb dessert options that are delicious and satisfying:

Recipe 1: Keto Chocolate Avocado Pudding

Ingredients:
- 2 ripe avocados
- 1/4 cup unsweetened cocoa powder
- 1/4 cup almond milk
- 1/4 cup of your favorite low-carb sweetener, or powdered erythritol
- 1 teaspoon vanilla extract
- A pinch of salt

Instructions:
1. Scoop the flesh from the avocados and place it in a blender or food processor.
2. Add cocoa powder, almond milk, powdered sweetener, vanilla extract, and a pinch of salt.
3. Blend until smooth and creamy.
4. Taste and adjust sweetness if needed.
5. Allow the dish to cool in the refrigerator for at least 30 minutes before serving.

Recipe 2: Sugar-Free Cheesecake Bites

Ingredients:
- 8 oz cream cheese, softened
- 1/4 cup of your favorite low-carb sweetener, or powdered erythritol
- 1 teaspoon vanilla extract
- Almond flour (for coating)

Instructions:
1. In a bowl, mix softened cream cheese, sweetener, and vanilla extract until smooth.
2. Roll the mixture into bite-sized balls.
3. Roll each ball in almond flour to coat.
4. Place on a tray and refrigerate for at least 1 hour before serving.

Recipe 3: Low-Carb Berry Parfait

Ingredients:
- Mixed berries (strawberries, blueberries, raspberries)
- 1 cup Greek yogurt (unsweetened or sweetened with a low-carb sweetener)
- Almond slices for topping
- Chia seeds (optional)

Instructions:
1. In a glass or bowl, layer Greek yogurt, mixed berries, and a sprinkle of chia seeds (if desired).
2. Repeat layers.
3. Top with almond slices for added crunch.

4. Serve chilled.

Tips for Low-Carb Desserts:

1. **Choose Sugar Substitutes:**
   - Utilize sugar substitutes like erythritol, stevia, or monk fruit to reduce carb content.

2. **Opt for Dark Chocolate:**
   - When incorporating chocolate, choose high-quality dark chocolate with lower sugar content.

3. **Experiment with Nut Flours:**
   - Almond flour and coconut flour can be great alternatives for traditional flours in low-carb desserts.

4. **Incorporate Berries:**
   - Berries are relatively low in carbs and can add natural sweetness.

5. **Mindful Portions:**
   - Enjoy desserts in moderation to stay within your carb goals.

Feel free to adjust these recipes to fit your taste preferences and dietary needs. These low-carb dessert options allow you to satisfy your sweet cravings while maintaining a lower carbohydrate intake.

Certainly! Here are three sweet treat recipes that are delightful and relatively easy to prepare:

Recipe 1: No-Bake Energy Bites

Ingredients:
- 1 cup old-fashioned oats
- Half a cup of nut butter (you can use peanut or almond butter).
- 1/3 cup honey or maple syrup
- 1/2 cup ground flaxseed
- 1/2 cup dark chocolate chips
- 1 teaspoon vanilla extract
- A pinch of salt

Instructions:
1. In a bowl, combine oats, nut butter, honey (or maple syrup), ground flaxseed, chocolate chips, vanilla extract, and a pinch of salt.
2. Mix until well combined.
3. Refrigerate the mixture for 15-30 minutes to make it easier to handle.
4. Take small portions and roll into bite-sized balls.
5. Place the energy bites on a tray and refrigerate for at least 1 hour before serving.

Recipe 2: Baked Cinnamon Apple Slices

Ingredients:
- 2 apples, thinly sliced

- 1 tablespoon melted butter or coconut oil
- 1 teaspoon ground cinnamon
- 1-2 teaspoons granulated erythritol or your preferred sweetener

Instructions:
1. Preheat the oven to 350°F (175°C).
2. In a bowl, toss apple slices with melted butter or coconut oil, ground cinnamon, and sweetener.
3. Arrange the slices on a baking sheet in a single layer.
4. Bake for 15-20 minutes or until apples are tender.
5. Serve warm as a cozy, low-carb dessert.

Recipe 3: Keto-Friendly Chocolate Avocado Mousse

Ingredients:
- 2 ripe avocados
- 1/4 cup unsweetened cocoa powder
- 1/4 cup almond milk
- 1/4 cup of your favorite low-carb sweetener or powdered erythritol
- 1 teaspoon vanilla extract
- A pinch of salt

Instructions:
1. Scoop the flesh from the avocados and place it in a blender or food processor.
2. Add cocoa powder, almond milk, powdered sweetener, vanilla extract, and a pinch of salt.

3. Blend until smooth and creamy.
4. Taste and adjust sweetness if needed.
5. Before serving, let the food cool for at least half an hour in the refrigerator.

Tips for Sweet Treats:

1. **Customize Sweetness:**
   - Adjust the sweetness level in recipes according to your taste preferences.

2. **Choose Quality Ingredients:**
   - Use high-quality chocolate and fresh fruits for enhanced flavor.

3. **Experiment with Flavors:**
   - Add spices like cinnamon or a dash of vanilla to enhance the flavor of your treats.

4. **Mindful Portions:**
   - Enjoy sweet treats in moderation to balance your overall diet.

Feel free to get creative and adjust these recipes to suit your dietary preferences. These sweet treats provide a satisfying and healthier alternative to traditional desserts.

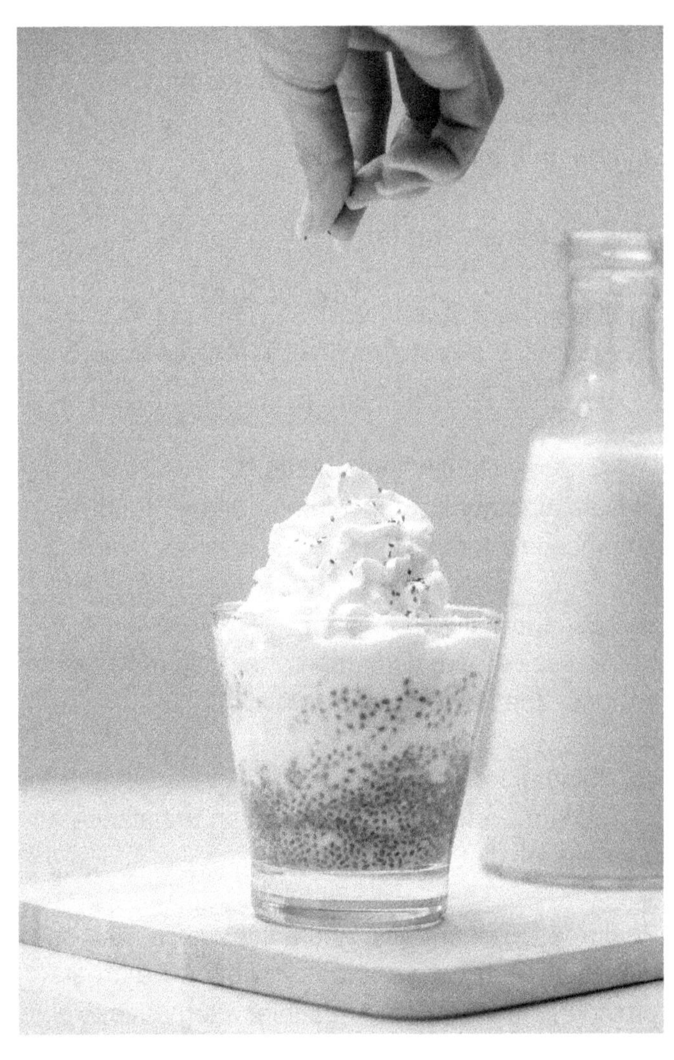

CHAPTER EIGHT

EATING OUT ON ATKINS

Eating out on the Atkins diet may require some thoughtful choices to stay within the low-carb guidelines. Here are some tips for making Atkins-friendly choices when dining out:

1. **Choose Grilled Proteins:**
   - Opt for grilled meats such as chicken, steak, or fish. Avoid breaded or battered options.

2. **Include Vegetables:**
   - Request non-starchy vegetables as side dishes. Examples include broccoli, spinach, asparagus, or a side salad.

3. **Skip the Bread and Grains:**
   - Ask for your meal without bread, croutons, or any grain-based sides.

4. **Be Wary of Sauces and Dressings:**
   - Check with the restaurant about sauces and dressings. Choose options without added sugars or opt for olive oil and vinegar.

5. **Choose Low-Carb Sides:**
   - If available, select low-carb side dishes like sautéed greens or cauliflower mash.

6. **Enjoy Eggs and Omelettes:**
   - Eggs are a great source of protein. Omelettes with veggies and cheese can be a satisfying choice.

7. **Gravitate Toward Seafood:**
   - Seafood is often low in carbs. Grilled or broiled fish can be a tasty and nutritious option.

8. **Customize Your Order:**
   - Don't hesitate to customize your order. Many restaurants are willing to accommodate dietary preferences.

9. **Beware of Hidden Carbs:**
   - Be cautious of hidden carbohydrates in marinades, dressings, and sauces. Ask for these on the side or choose options with minimal added sugars.

10. **Hydrate:**
    - Water or other unsweetened drinks will help you stay hydrated. Be cautious of high-sugar drinks.

11. **Ask Questions:**
    - Don't be afraid to ask your server questions about the menu and how dishes are prepared. This helps you make informed choices.

12. **Avoid Fried Foods:**

- Batter or flour are frequently used to coat fried dishes. Instead, go for baked, grilled, or broiled options.

13. **Consider Portion Sizes:**
   - Pay attention to portion sizes. Some restaurant servings can be larger than necessary, and you can ask for a half portion or take leftovers home.

14. **Plan Ahead:**
   - If possible, check the restaurant's menu online beforehand to plan your low-carb choices.

Remember, flexibility is key, and making mindful choices can help you enjoy dining out while following the Atkins diet. Don't hesitate to communicate your dietary preferences with the restaurant staff to ensure a more enjoyable and compliant dining experience.

MAKING WISE MENU CHOICES

Making wise menu choices, especially when following a specific dietary plan like Atkins, involves considering the composition of dishes and selecting options that align with your nutritional goals. Here are some general guidelines for making wise menu choices:

1. **Focus on Protein:**

- Prioritize dishes rich in protein. Opt for lean meats, fish, poultry, eggs, or vegetarian protein sources.

2. **Choose Non-Starchy Vegetables:**
   - Include non-starchy vegetables as a significant portion of your meal. Leafy greens, broccoli, cauliflower, zucchini, and bell peppers are a few examples.

3. **Limit Carbohydrates:**
   - Be cautious with high-carb items like bread, pasta, rice, and potatoes. Consider alternatives such as cauliflower rice, zucchini noodles, or lettuce wraps.

4. **Opt for Grilled or Baked Preparations:**
   - Choose grilled, baked, or broiled dishes over fried or breaded options to minimize unnecessary carbs.

5. **Watch Sauces and Dressings:**
   - Be mindful of sauces and dressings, as they can contain added sugars. Ask for dressings on the side or choose vinaigrettes made with olive oil.

6. **Customize Your Order:**
   - Don't hesitate to customize your meal. Ask for substitutions or modifications to fit your dietary preferences.

7. **Beware of Hidden Sugars:**

- Watch out for hidden sugars, especially in condiments, marinades, and sauces. Opt for items without added sugars.

8. **Portion Control:**
   - Pay attention to portion sizes. Restaurants often serve larger portions, so consider sharing or saving part of your meal for later.

9. **Hydrate with Water:**
   - Drink water with your meal instead of sugary beverages. Drinking water helps regulate your appetite in addition to keeping you hydrated.

10. **Include Healthy Fats:**
    - Incorporate sources of healthy fats, such as avocados, olive oil, or nuts, to add flavor and satiety to your meal.

11. **Scan the Menu Ahead of Time:**
    - If possible, review the menu online before going to the restaurant. This allows you to plan your order and make informed choices.

12. **Choose Whole, Unprocessed Foods:**
    - Opt for whole, unprocessed foods rather than heavily processed options. Fresh, whole ingredients are generally better for your health.

13. **Consider Your Individual Needs:**

- Take into account your specific dietary needs and preferences. Different people may have different responses to certain foods.

14. **Listen to Your Body:**
   - Observe the signals of hunger and fullness your body sends you. Stop eating when you're satisfied, not overly full.

Making wise menu choices is about balance, awareness, and choosing foods that align with your health and dietary goals. By staying mindful of your choices and being aware of the nutritional content of dishes, you can enjoy meals that support your well-being.

TIPS FOR DINING OUT SUCCESSFULLY

Dining out successfully while following a specific dietary plan, such as Atkins, requires some strategic planning. Here are tips to help you navigate restaurants and make healthier choices:

1. **Review the Menu in Advance:**
   - Check the restaurant's menu online beforehand to identify low-carb options. This allows you to make informed choices and avoid feeling pressured when ordering.

2. **Choose Protein-Rich Options:**

- Prioritize dishes that are rich in protein, such as grilled chicken, fish, steak, or vegetarian protein sources. Protein helps keep you satisfied.

3. **Include Non-Starchy Vegetables:**
   - Opt for non-starchy vegetables as side dishes or as part of your main course. These include leafy greens, broccoli, cauliflower, and asparagus.

4. **Customize Your Order:**
   - Don't hesitate to customize your meal. Ask for substitutions, adjustments, or modifications to make the dish align with your dietary preferences.

5. **Watch Portion Sizes:**
   - Be mindful of portion sizes, as restaurant servings can be larger than necessary. Think about bringing leftovers home or splitting an entree.

6. **Beware of Hidden Carbs:**
   - Watch out for hidden carbohydrates in marinades, dressings, and sauces. Ask for these on the side or choose options with minimal added sugars.

7. **Choose Grilled or Baked Preparations:**
   - Opt for grilled, baked, or broiled dishes over fried or breaded options to minimize unnecessary carbohydrates.

8. **Be Mindful of Sauces and Dressings:**

- Watch out for hidden carbohydrates in marinades, dressings, and sauces. Consider using olive oil and vinegar for salads.

9. **Stay Hydrated:**
   - To stay hydrated, sip water during your meal. Refrain from sugar-filled drinks and cut back on booze.

10. **Plan for Low-Carb Sides:**
    - Request non-starchy vegetable sides, and if available, choose options like sautéed spinach, Brussels sprouts, or asparagus.

11. **Communicate Dietary Preferences:**
    - Communicate clearly with your server about your dietary preferences and any specific needs you have. Most restaurants are willing to accommodate.

12. **Avoid Bread Baskets:**
    - Politely decline the bread basket to avoid unnecessary carb intake before your meal arrives.

13. **Choose Simple Preparations:**
    - Opt for dishes with simple ingredient lists to minimize the likelihood of hidden carbs.

14. **Consider Salad Options:**
    - Salads are a fantastic low-carb option. Ensure they include protein, healthy fats, and non-starchy vegetables.

15. **Practice Moderation:**
   - Enjoy your meal in moderation. Focus on savoring the flavors and listening to your body's hunger cues.

Remember, dining out is about enjoying the experience, and with thoughtful choices, you can adhere to your dietary preferences while still savoring delicious meals. Don't be afraid to communicate your needs and make adjustments to suit your plan.

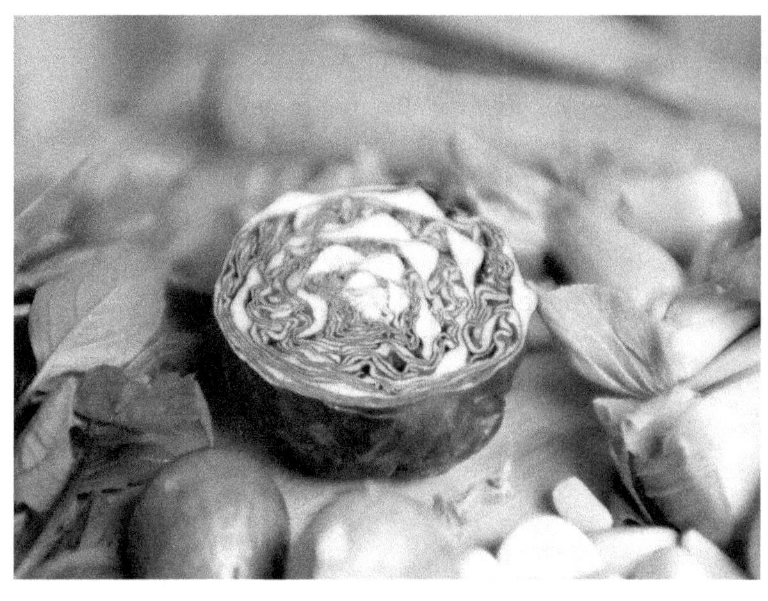

CHAPTER NINE

TROUBLESHOOTING AND COMMON QUESTIONS

Certainly! Here are some troubleshooting tips and common questions that individuals following the Atkins diet might encounter:

Troubleshooting:

1. **Not Seeing Results:**
   - Make sure you are monitoring your carbohydrate intake correctly. Hidden carbs or incorrect portion sizes may impact your progress.

2. **Feeling Fatigued:**
   - Electrolyte balance and proper hydration are essential. Consider increasing your water intake and incorporating electrolyte-rich foods or supplements.

3. **Plateauing:**
   - Plateaus can happen. Review your diet for hidden carbs, reassess your portion sizes, and consider incorporating more variety in your meals.

4. **Digestive Issues:**
   - If experiencing digestive discomfort, ensure you are getting enough fiber from non-starchy

vegetables. Gradually increase fiber intake to allow your body to adjust.

5. **Sugar Cravings:**
   - Sugar cravings may persist initially. Focus on satisfying alternatives, such as berries, and be patient as your body adjusts to reduced sugar intake.

6. **Lack of Variety:**
   - To keep your meals interesting, experiment with different ingredients and recipes. A lack of variety may contribute to boredom with your eating plan.

Common Questions:

1. **Can I Have Fruit?**
   - Yes, but in moderation. Berries (strawberries, blueberries, raspberries) are lower in carbs. To avoid going over your daily carbohydrate allowance, watch meal sizes.

2. **How Do I Handle Social Situations?**
   - Plan ahead by checking restaurant menus and making wise choices. Communicate your dietary needs with friends or family to ensure supportive environments.

3. **Is Alcohol Allowed?**
   - Some low-carb alcoholic beverages (like dry wine or spirits) can be consumed in moderation. Be mindful of mixers and added sugars.

4. **Can I Have Dairy?**
   - Yes, many dairy products are low in carbs. Opt for full-fat options and be cautious with flavored varieties that may contain added sugars.

5. **How Long Should I Stay in Induction?**
   - The induction phase typically lasts 2 weeks. However, individual responses vary. Progress to subsequent phases as you feel comfortable and see results.

6. **Can I Follow Atkins as a Vegetarian or Vegan?**
   - Yes, it's possible. Focus on plant-based protein sources, non-starchy vegetables, and healthy fats. Consider plant-based protein supplements if needed.

7. **Do I Need to Count Calories?**
   - While not mandatory, some individuals find calorie tracking helpful for weight management. Pay attention to the caliber of the meals you choose.

8. **Is Exercise Necessary?**
   - Exercise is beneficial for overall health. While not mandatory for the Atkins diet, incorporating physical activity can enhance weight loss and well-being.

For individualized guidance, always speak with a medical professional or a licensed dietitian. Adjustments may be necessary based on individual health conditions and goals.

ADDRESSING CHALLENGES

Addressing challenges while following the Atkins diet involves understanding common hurdles and implementing strategies to overcome them. Here are ways to tackle some challenges:

Challenge: **Sugar Cravings

Strategy:
   - **Choose Sweet Alternatives:** Incorporate low-carb sweet treats like berries or sugar-free desserts to satisfy cravings.
   - **Gradual Reduction:** Gradually reduce sugar intake to allow your taste buds to adjust over time.
   - **Stay Hydrated:** Sometimes, dehydration can be mistaken for hunger. Drink water when cravings strike.

Challenge: **Social Situations and Dining Out

Strategy:
   - **Plan Ahead:** Check restaurant menus in advance and plan your order.

- **Communication:** Communicate your dietary needs with friends or family to create supportive environments.
- **BYO Snacks:** Bring low-carb snacks to social events to ensure you have suitable options.

Challenge: **Lack of Variety in Meals**

Strategy:
- **Explore New Recipes:** Experiment with new ingredients and recipes to keep meals interesting.
- **Rotate Foods:** Rotate different protein sources, vegetables, and fats to add variety to your diet.
- **Spice It Up:** Use herbs and spices to enhance flavors without adding carbs.

Challenge: **Plateau in Weight Loss**

Strategy:
- **Reassess Portion Sizes:** Double-check portion sizes to ensure you're not unintentionally consuming more carbs than intended.
- **Increase Activity:** Incorporate more physical activity to boost metabolism.
- **Dietary Variety:** Introduce new foods and adjust your macronutrient ratios to avoid a dietary plateau.

Challenge: **Feeling Fatigued or Low Energy**

Strategy:

- **Electrolyte Balance:** Ensure adequate hydration and consider electrolyte-rich foods or supplements.
- **Adjust Macros:** Tweak your macronutrient ratios to find the balance that provides sustained energy.
- **Adequate Calories:** Ensure you're consuming enough calories to meet your energy needs.

Challenge: **Social Pressure and Criticism**

Strategy:
- **Educate Others:** Share information about the Atkins diet and its benefits with those who may not be familiar.
- **Stick to Your Plan:** Politely decline offers of food that don't align with your dietary goals.
- **Express Your Goals:** Clearly communicate your health and weight loss goals to others.

Challenge: **Digestive Issues**

Strategy:
- **Gradual Increase in Fiber:** If increasing fiber, do so gradually to allow your digestive system to adapt.
- **Hydration:** Ensure sufficient water intake to help with digestion.
- **Probiotics:** Consider incorporating probiotic-rich foods or supplements for gut health.

Recall that every person's experience is unique, and it's critical to pay attention to your body. If challenges persist or are concerning, consult with a healthcare professional or a registered dietitian for personalized guidance.

FAQ'S AND SOLUTIONS

Certainly! Here are some frequently asked questions (FAQs) about the Atkins diet along with solutions:

Q1: Can I have fruits on the Atkins diet?

Solution:
   - Yes, but in moderation. Opt for lower-carb fruits like berries (strawberries, blueberries, raspberries) and control portion sizes to stay within your daily carb limit.

Q2: How do I deal with sugar cravings?

Solution:
   - Choose sugar alternatives like stevia or erythritol.
   - Satisfy cravings with small portions of dark chocolate or sugar-free desserts.
   - Gradually reduce sugar intake to allow your taste buds to adjust.

Q3: Can I follow Atkins as a vegetarian or vegan?

Solution:
- Yes, it's possible. Give priority to plant-based protein sources such as beans, tempeh, and tofu.
- Include non-starchy vegetables, healthy fats, and consider plant-based protein supplements if needed.

Q4: How do I handle social situations or dining out?

Solution:
- Examine restaurant menus to make advance plans.
- Communicate your dietary needs with friends or family to create supportive environments.
- Choose protein-rich options with non-starchy vegetables when dining out.

Q5: Is exercise necessary on the Atkins diet?

Solution:
- Exercise is beneficial for overall health but not mandatory for the diet.
- Incorporate physical activity for added health benefits and weight management.

Q6: How long should I stay in the Induction phase?

Solution:
  - The induction phase typically lasts 2 weeks. Progress to subsequent phases as you feel comfortable and see results.

Q7: Can I consume alcohol on the Atkins diet?

Solution:
  - Some low-carb alcoholic beverages (dry wine, spirits) can be consumed in moderation.
  - Be cautious of mixers and added sugars in cocktails.

Q8: What if I hit a weight loss plateau?

Solution:
  - Reassess portion sizes and track your food accurately.
  - Introduce new foods and adjust macronutrient ratios.
  - Step up your exercise to speed up your metabolism.

Q9: How do I handle digestive issues?

Solution:
  - Gradually increase fiber intake to allow your digestive system to adapt.
  - Ensure sufficient hydration.
  - Consider incorporating probiotic-rich foods or supplements for gut health.

Q10: How can I add variety to my meals?

Solution:
   - Explore new recipes and ingredients.
   - Rotate different protein sources, vegetables, and fats.
   - Use herbs and spices to enhance flavors without adding carbs.

Remember, individual responses may vary, and it's essential to tailor the diet to your specific needs. If you have concerns or specific health conditions, consult with a healthcare professional or a registered dietitian for personalized advice.

CONCLUSION

In conclusion, embarking on the Atkins diet is a journey toward improved health, sustainable weight management, and a redefined relationship with food. As you navigate the different phases, from Induction to Maintenance, keep in mind the following key takeaways:

1. **Personalization is Key:**
   - Tailor the Atkins approach to suit your individual needs, preferences, and health goals. A person's ideal fit can not always be what suits another.

2. **Gradual Progression:**
   - Embrace the gradual progression between phases. Each stage serves a purpose, whether it's kickstarting weight loss in Induction or finding a balanced maintenance plan.

3. **Nutrient-Rich Choices:**
   - Focus on nutrient-rich foods, including lean proteins, healthy fats, and non-starchy vegetables. This not only supports your dietary goals but also ensures you're getting essential nutrients.

4. **Mindful Eating:**
   - Cultivate mindfulness in your eating habits. Pay attention to hunger and fullness cues, savor the flavors of your meals, and build a positive relationship with food.

5. **Strategic Carb Management:**

- Manage your carbohydrate intake strategically. Be aware of hidden carbs, gradually introduce more carbs during the phases, and find the balance that works for your body.

6. **Lifestyle Integration:**

- View the Atkins diet as a lifestyle rather than a temporary fix. Embrace the principles of balanced nutrition, regular exercise, and long-term well-being.

7. **Celebrating Achievements:**

- Acknowledge and celebrate your achievements, both on and off the scale. Non-scale victories such as increased energy, improved mood, and enhanced confidence are integral to your success.

8. **Flexibility and Adaptability:**

- Stay flexible and adaptable. Life may present challenges, and your ability to adjust while staying committed to your goals will contribute to your long-term success.

9. **Support System:**

- Surround yourself with a supportive network. Whether it's friends, family, or fellow Atkins participants, having a support system can provide motivation, encouragement, and shared experiences.

10. **Continued Learning:**

- Stay informed and continue to learn about nutrition, health, and the science behind the Atkins diet. You can make decisions that are best for your wellbeing when you are well-informed.

11. **Consultation with Professionals:**
- Always consult with healthcare professionals or registered dietitians, especially if you have pre-existing health conditions. Their guidance ensures that your dietary choices align with your overall health needs.

As you embark on or continue your Atkins journey, remember that it's a process of self-discovery and positive transformation. Embrace the opportunity to cultivate a healthier, more vibrant version of yourself. Here's to your continued success and well-being!

CELEBRATING YOUR ACHIEVEMENT

Congratulations on reaching a milestone or achieving a goal! Celebrating your achievements is an important part of recognizing your hard work and dedication. Here are some ideas for commemorating your achievement:

1. **Reflect on Your Journey:**

- Consider your path for a moment. Consider the progress you've made, the challenges you've overcome, and the personal growth you've experienced.

2. **Reward Yourself:**
   - Treat yourself to a well-deserved reward. Whether it's a small indulgence, a favorite activity, or something you've been looking forward to, celebrate with a special treat.

3. **Share Your Success:**
   - Share your achievement with friends, family, or a supportive community. Their positive feedback and congratulations can amplify the joy of your success.

4. **Capture the Moment:**
   - Take photos or create a journal entry to capture the moment. Documenting your achievements allows you to revisit and appreciate your progress in the future.

5. **Plan a Celebration Meal:**
   - Enjoy a celebratory meal that aligns with your dietary choices. Select meals that fill you up and make you feel wonderful.

6. **Pamper Yourself:**
   - Treat yourself to a spa day, a massage, or any form of self-care that helps you relax and unwind. Honor your successes by looking for yourself.

7. **Set New Goals:**
   - Consider setting new goals or milestones to continue your journey. Having future objectives keeps you motivated and excited about what lies ahead.

8. **Express Gratitude:**
   - Take a moment to express gratitude for the support you've received, the lessons you've learned, and the strength that carried you through. Gratitude enhances the positive impact of your achievements.

9. **Create a Memory:**
   - Create a lasting memory associated with your accomplishment. Whether it's a symbolic item, a framed photo, or a written note, having a tangible reminder can be meaningful.

10. **Host a Celebration Event:**
    - If applicable, host a small gathering with friends and family to celebrate together. Share the joy of your achievement with those who have supported you.

11. **Give Back:**
    - Pay it forward by contributing to a cause or community that holds significance for you. Giving back can be a meaningful way to celebrate your success.

Remember, celebrating your achievements is not only about recognizing the endpoint but also acknowledging the journey. Embrace the positive energy, be proud of your accomplishments, and use this celebration as fuel for your continued success.